BIBLICAL PRAYER

AGAINST

SICKNESS AND DISEASES

By Tella Olayeri

08023583168

Email; tellaolayeri@gmail.com
Website www.tellaolayeri.com

US Contact
Ruth Jack
14 Milewood Road
Verbank
N.Y.12585
U.S.A. +19176428989

APPRECIATION

I give special appreciation to my wife **MRS NGOZI OLAYERI** for her assistance in ensuring that this book is published and our children that play around us to encourage us day and night.

Also, this manuscript wouldn't have seen the light of the day, if not for the spiritual encouragement I gathered from my father in the Lord, **Dr. D.K. OLUKOYA** who served as spiritual mirror that brightens my hope to explore my calling (Evangelism).

We shall all reap our blessings in heaven but the battle to make heaven is not over, until it is won.

PREFACE

The Holy Bible is a book loaded with words of salvation, faith, encouragement, obedience, victory, love, mercy, thanksgiving, trial, good health and many others. God wants us to have hope in what we do or pass through. He is there for us all the time.

God did not create us to be consumed by any form of sickness, disease or infirmity. He said we shall have control and dominion over everything created. In the beginning there wasn't anything like sickness or disease, until we sin against God.

But then God makes provision for us to live long life, if we follow simple rule to distance ourselves from sin and worship him. The Lord said, **"If you listen carefully to the voice of the LORD your God and do what is right in his eyes, if you pay attention to his commands and keep all his decrees, I will not bring on you any of the diseases I brought on the Egyptians, for I am the LORD, who heals you" Exodus 15:26.**

Based on this promise, we should not suffer any sickness, disease or infirmity. But as a result of our sin God allow them to happen. All is not lost, as window of prayer is open to us. With prayer we overcome problems, deficiencies, disease and sickness unhurt. The book of **Psalm 91:7 says "A thousand may fall at your side, ten thousand at your right hand, but it will not come near you."** Definitely, sickness and disease may strike, it will not come near you, only shall you witness it with your eyes.

This book is purely biblically based prayer book with chapters based on bible passages. The pillar and strength of the book is promise of God on healing and deliverance. It is a spiritual loaded health prayer book every home should have.

GOOD NEWS!!!

My audiobook is now available, to get one visit acx.com and search **"Tella Olayeri."**

Brethren, to be loaded and reloaded visit: *amazon.com/author/tellaolayeri* for a full spiritual sojourn for my books.

Thanks.

PREVIOUS PUBLICATIONS OF THE AUTHOR

1. *Fire for Fire Prayer Book Part 1*
2. *Fire for Fire Prayer Book Part 2*
3. *My Marriage Shall Not Break*
4. *Prayer for Pregnant Women*
5. *Prayer for the Fruit of the Womb*
6. *Children Deliverance*
7. *Prayer for Youths and Teenagers*
8. *Prayer for Singles*
9. *Victory over Satanic House Part 1*
10. *Victory over Satanic House Part 2*
11. *I Shall Excel*
12. *Atomic Prayers that Destroy Witchcraft Powers and Silence Enemies*
13. *Goliath at the Gate of Marriage*
14. *Deliverance from Spirit of Dogs*
15. *Naked Warriors*
16. *Prayer Against Sex in the Dream*
17. *Strange Women! Leave My Husband Alone*
18. *Dangerous Prayer against Strange Women*
19. *630 Acidic Prayer Points*
20. *Power to Retain Job and Excel in Office*
21. *Warfare in the Office*
22. *Command the Year*
23. *Deliverance Prayer for First Born*
24. *800 Deliverance Prayer for First Born Part Two*
25. *Prayer for Good Health and Divine Healing*
26. *Prayer against Untimely Death.*
27. *Dictionary of Dreams*

Table of Contents

CHAPTER 1

PRAYER AGAINST INFIRMITIES AND DISEASES

We need God more than ever. We have seen the miracles he performed and we believe he can do more. **"For nothing is impossible with God" Luke 1:17**. The sick bed is not our portion as children of God. We trust him, we believe in him. We have assurance in his healing power. May the grace of the Lord Almighty locate us wherever we are, amen.

Brethren the fact of the matter is, no sickness shall overtake you. You shall not be stranded in this crucial time. You shall experience smooth acceleration even in the midst of economic and health recession battling the world. There is this strong assurance, you shall overtake and possess your possession; and be of good health. The Lord shall keep you safe. Amen

Our God, Yahweh, is the creator and all-powerful God. He knows the beginning and the ending. He knows our health history; he knows there is infirmity and disease to contend with. He is bigger than all our fears and wiser than all the troubles ahead. Without him, we are helpless and would never get the healing we need.

Our call to God; is to stretch forth his healing arm and end the battle of ill-health troubling our soul. Our Lord Jesus Christ; heals anytime of the day. Infirmity and disease is but a child play to him. He is never tired. The bible records it. **"That evening after sunset the people brought to Jesus all the sick and demon possessed. The whole town gathered at the door, and Jesus healed many who had various diseases." Mark 1:32-34.**

In medical circle meanings are given to infirmity and disease. They define infirmity as the quality or state of being weak or ill especially because of old age. Also, they say, it's a disease or illness that usually last for a long time. At times, patient may have an unsound mind, and or, being sick. But Jesus, don't believe in definition or prescriptions, but in the Word and word of the mouth. He commands and heaven hears, while result is achieved. When Simon's mother-in law was in bed with fever, and they told him, he only went there held her hand out of bed, and she was healed Mark 1:30-31. Today, our LORD shall hold hands of every sick ones out of bed. Amen

The miracle Jesus performed were uncountable during his time, and he is still doing it. **"Jesus went throughout Galilee, teaching in their synagogues, preaching the good news of the kingdom, and healing every disease and sickness among the people." Mathew 4:23.**

What Jesus needs is your faith and believe. He hates definition of disease or fear of, it can't be healed or cure. Yes, doctors will say there are four types of disease; namely *infectious diseases, deficiency diseases, hereditary diseases and physiological diseases.* All these are manmade definition, not God. When Jesus came to the scene the disease will vanish. At the mention of his name, all knees shall bow.

Jesus doesn't apply vaccine as applied to chicken pox or measles. He doesn't follow symptoms or signs of disease. All he does is to heal. It is that supernatural healing power we shall ask for today. Jesus doesn't want to know how you contact the disease. What he understands is healing. Jesus doesn't want to know your immune system, whether it is weak or not. By laying his hand upon you, or hold you, speak to you, your healing is imminent.

It is time you cry to God. Raise your voice to the Lord. Though doctors, have spoken, we depend on the word of the Almighty. Your faith shouldn't be in the utterance of men, but on his eternal grace. Ask for his healing. Let's ask for his healing over the world, our self, and family. We pray that the Lord Almighty shall do more than what the doctors can do. May the Lord Almighty heal our body today, in Jesus name, Amen.

Now let's pray.

PRAYER POINTS

1. I thank you Lord for your mercy and love for me, in the name of Jesus.
2. I thank my God for he shall heal me of every disease and infirmity in the name of Jesus.
3. I thank my God, his hand of healing shall not pass me bye, in the name of Jesus.
4. I thank my God, who will stand by me, throughout this prayer, in the name of Jesus.
5. Lord Jesus, lay hand of forgiveness upon me, in the name of Jesus.
6. Lord Jesus forgive me of sins I commit before, now and any I may have in mind so that I can have rest.

7. Lord Jesus, I am a sinner, have mercy upon me.
8. Lord Jesus, open door of forgiveness for me, by your power.
9. O Lord, let my petition be accepted before you, in the name of Jesus.
10. Woe unto powers that direct my steps to sin, in the name of Jesus.
11. Blood of Jesus, set me free from disease and infirmity, in the name of Jesus.
12. I drink blood of Jesus to cleanse me of any impurity deposited in my body, in the name of Jesus.
13. I cover myself with blood of Jesus against diseases and sickness, in the name of Jesus.
14. I soak myself in the pool blood of Jesus.
15. I surround myself with blood of Jesus.
16. Holy Spirit, direct my step to palace of deliverance that eliminate sickness and disease, in the name of Jesus.
17. Holy Spirit, guide me with heavenly support to overcome health issues of life.
18. Holy Ghost power, give me strength to pray and excel in life in the name of Jesus.
19. Holy Spirit, touch my soul, spirit and body, in the name of Jesus.

20. Holy Spirit Divine, wear me with garment of healing, in the name of Jesus.
21. Every arrow of disease fired against me from the pit of hell backfire, in the name of Jesus.
22. Sickbed assigned for me in the spirit, break to pieces and catch fire, in the name of Jesus.
23. Satanic doctor assign to finalize my health for negative purpose, my life is not your candidate, die, in the name of Jesus.
24. Satanic nurse waiting for my arrival at dark hospital you are a failure, die, and rise no more, in the name of Jesus.
25. Diseases assign for me in the spirit, expire, in the name of Jesus.
26. O Lord, silence every virus assign to eliminate me and my household, in the name of Jesus.
27. Evil doctor report about me in the spirit, catch fire and roast to ashes, in the name of Jesus.
28. O Lord, let your healing come mightily upon my family, in the name of Jesus.
29. O Lord, let your healing come mightily upon my nation and the world, in the name of Jesus.
30. Lord Jesus, I need you more than ever, come and heal me, in the name of Jesus.
31. Satanic pastor, satanic Alfas, assign to attack me with sickness, carry your load, in the name of Jesus.

32. Nothing is impossible with you O Lord, make every impossibility in my life possible, in the name of Jesus.

33. Every satanic arrangement to infect me with infirmity at early age scatter in the name of Jesus.

34. Satanic arrangement to attack me with sickness from the pit of hell, scatter, in the name of Jesus.

35. Satanic arrangement to attack me with disease, scatter in the name of Jesus.

36. Sickbed is not my portion, I shall not be allotted one in the name of Jesus.

37. Every sickness assign to overtake me shall fail, in the name of Jesus.

38. Ancient of days, heal me in and out, in the name of Jesus.

39. I overcome effect of economic recession assign to destroy my health life, in the name of Jesus.

40. I shall overtake and possess my possession in the name of Jesus.

41. My health history shall not be polluted or destroyed, in the name of Jesus.

42. Ambulance assign for emergency, I am not your candidate, catch fire and roast to ashes, in the name of Jesus.

43. Evil caterer assign to feed me with satanic food, my life is not your candidate, die, in the name of Jesus.
44. Evil food that infects one with disease served to me in the dream, catch fire and roast to ashes, in the name of Jesus.
45. Every disease and infirmity assign to consume me, die in the name of Jesus.
46. O Lord, pull down and destroy every trouble ahead of me, in the name of Jesus.
47. O Lord stretch forth your healing arm and end the battle of ill-health assign to trouble me, in the name of Jesus.
48. Whatever the name of any sickness or disease, it shall not be my portion, in the name of Jesus.
49. Unsound mind created for me in the spirit, expire, in the name of Jesus.
50. My environment, receive healing, in the name of Jesus.
51. Lord Jesus, single me out for deliverance and heal me in the name of Jesus.
52. Lord Jesus, feed me with your word that liberates, in the name of Jesus.
53. Products of disease, fever, malaria, measles are not my portion in the name of Jesus.
54. I anchor myself to the healing name of Jesus, in the name of Jesus.

55. What doctors cannot do to heal me, my God shall heal me perfectly well, in the name of Jesus.

56. I wear garment of eternal grace of God, in the name of Jesus.

57. Though doctors may speak, the word of the Lord, that says I am healed is final, therefore, I am healed, in the name of Jesus.

58. Satanic clock regulating my health, break to pieces in the name of Jesus.

59. Heavenly fire; radiate round me, and kill every bacterial and virus keeping me in bondage, in the name of Jesus.

60. O Lord, sanitize my house from danger, in the name of Jesus.

61. Every trace of disease in my lineage, expire, in the name of Jesus.

62. Powers of darkness, you shall harvest failure in your pursuit against me, in the name of Jesus.

63. O Lord, give me perfect healing in the name of Jesus.

64. Every evil clinical report about me, expire, in the name of Jesus.

65. Heavenly health workers, take care of me and heal me in the name of Jesus.

66. Wound in my body in the spirit; be healed, in the name of Jesus.

67. Total healing from above, be my portion in the name of Jesus.
68. Every pain in my body, receive divine healing, in the name of Jesus.
69. Workers of iniquities shall fail woefully concerning my life, in the name of Jesus.
70. I am free from every form of sickness or disease, in the name of Jesus.

CHAPTER 2

PRAYER OF PROTECTION USING PSALM 91

The book of Psalm 91 is awesome, promising and fire loaded with truth and artillery of words. When all hope is lost, ensure you read this assurance chapter of the bible.

The assurance is based on the premise you must dwell in the Lord, meaning come to HIM and surrender with faith. The shadow of the Lord is powerful, protective and real. The shadow of the Lord serves as protection from every disease and infirmity. In his shadow you are protected, with loaded joy, while fear disappears.

With total submission, walk unto the Lord for salvation and healing. Make him your personal Lord and savior. Don't doubt his love and power. He is our refuge and fortress against all manner of sickness and disease. When you say someone is your refuge, you mean he can do all things, when you say he is your fortress, it means you never doubt his power to give you rest. In his fortress, sickness is zero, infirmity is none existent, and disease never exists.

He will save you from every snare and fowler. He is battle ready to make you independent of infirmity and disease. The assurance is hundred percent. No deadly pestilence can devour or kill you in as much you dwell in his fortress. No virus shall lay hand on you to devour you.

The Lord will cover you with his feather. This feather is covered with fire of deliverance and hope. No matter your condition, in as much you run unto him, you are saved. When hen sees enemy, she opens her feather for her children, for protection. If hen do this, what then is difficult for God to do for us, if we find our way under the protection of his feather?

In the day and night, you are protected from fear and attack of disease and infirmity. At night, when you are asleep, no terror shall consume you, in the day no arrow shall send you to early grave. The Lord is there for you. Run unto him now, he is the one that gives 24/7 protection against virus attack, sickness, disease, and infirmity.

The Bible makes us to understand that pestilences are evil powers that destroy at night. They kill at will at night. I pray it shall not be your portion. The plague kills at day, but it shall not consume you in the order of Egyptians. Every, pestilence and plague assign to consume you shall fail woefully, in the name of Jesus. **"A thousand may fall at your side, ten thousand at your right hand, but it will not come near you. You will only observe with your eyes and see punishment of the wicked." Psalm 91:7-8.**

This is undiluted assurance of God for you. Believe in HIM only. No harm that walks or fly about shall consume you. You are save in the hands of the Lord Almighty, with his Angels all around to guide you from attack of pestilence, plague, virus, disease or infirmity. No matter their nature in form of demonic lion or serpent, the Lord shall make you to overcome them all.

With God, your health is guaranteed. No sickness or disease shall come near you. Fast and pray. Take precaution of hygiene. Even as you fast and pray, take your bath, clean up your surrounding; and follow every step that supports life.

The monster called death shall not come near you once you are under the shadow of the Most High God. He is your creator. He knows your chemistry and biological formation. He heals, save and strengthen soul. You are God's candidate. No arrow of darkness shall consume you. No biological weapon shall send you to early grave. No disease shall block your respiratory organ. No disease shall kill you. No disease shall eat you and render you useless. No announcement of death shall happen in your house, in the name of Jesus.

Because the Lord loves you, He will do everything to protect you from every plague and pestilence. You will call upon him now in prayer, surely he will answer you. The Lord is waiting for you, open your mouth wide and pray unto HIM. He is Almighty, so mighty that no sickness or disease can stop HIM.

Now let's pray;

PRAYER POINTS

1. O Lord my father, forgive me every sin that stands on my way against your favor and love for me, in the name of Jesus.
2. O Lord, forgive me every sin in my life that invites sickness to my life in the name of Jesus.
3. Every cup of sin in my hand, break to pieces, in the name of Jesus.
4. Sin that invite death to life, tormenting me, O Lord let it stop now in the name of Jesus.

5. Every sin that stands between me and my creator be nullified by the power in the blood of Jesus.
6. O Lord, I thank you for your protection upon me, in the name of Jesus.
7. I thank you Lord, for you shall not surrender me to the hands of untimely death, in the name of Jesus.
8. I thank my God, the only one that can't be killed with sickness or disease, in the name of Jesus.
9. O Lord, I thank you for sparing my life, to this day, in the name of Jesus.
10. I thank my God, for his grace upon my life, in the name of Jesus.
11. Blood of Jesus, cover me, protect me and strengthen me, in the name of Jesus.
12. Blood of Jesus, flow in my life, give me new birth, in the name of Jesus.
13. I drink blood of Jesus, to cleanse me of every infirmity, sickness or disease in the name of Jesus.
14. Blood of Jesus, enter my vein and flush out every sickness in me, in the name of Jesus.
15. Spirit of God, make way for me to live and be old in the Lord, in the name of Jesus.

16. Holy Spirit, scatter and destroy plague of disease in my vicinity in the name of Jesus.

17. Holy Spirit Divine, protect me by fire, in the name of Jesus.

18. Holy Spirit, teach me how to pray and receive answer, in the name of Jesus.

19. Heavenly protection, take over my life, in the name of Jesus.

20. Lord Jesus, show love unto me today as I raise my voice unto you today, in the name of Jesus.

21. Angels that rescue souls from untimely death, rescue my soul today, in the name of Jesus.

22. Angels of protection in the heavenly, come down today, and rescue me from the jaw of sickness and disease, in the name of Jesus.

23. O Lord, I call upon you, answer me by fire, in the name of Jesus.

24. O Lord, you promise, you will be with me in time of trouble, scatter and destroy every work of darkness in my life, in the name of Jesus.

25. O Lord, command your angel to devour and destroy every disease in the air around me and my household, in the name of Jesus.

26. Every deadly pestilence assign to kill me, die, in the name of Jesus.

27. Deadly food, catch fire and roast to ashes, in the name of Jesus.

28. Every chain of disease and sickness in my life, break, in the name of Jesus.
29. Fire feather of God, protect me by fire, in the name of Jesus.
30. O Lord, let your feather of deliverance protect me from flying disease of infirmity, in the name of Jesus.
31. O Lord, cover me with your feather of glory and favour that which will stand me out anywhere I go, in the name of Jesus.
32. O Lord, feed me with food of long life and prosperity, in the name of Jesus.
33. O Lord, I run to your shelter, receive me and protect me from evil arrow, in the name of Jesus.
34. O Lord, let your faithfulness be my food, in the name of Jesus.
35. O Lord, let your shield give me protection from arrow of disease, in the name of Jesus.
36. Snare of sickness and disease warming up to consume me and my family, catch fire and roast to ashes, in the name of Jesus.
37. Every fear of terror of the night, die, in the name of Jesus.
38. Disease and infirmity, my life is not your candidate, die, in the name of Jesus.

39. Every pestilence that stalks in darkness, die, in the name of Jesus.

40. Every plague released in the spirit to consume me and my household, die, in the name of Jesus.

41. Witchcraft powers that manufacture weapons of death, die with your weapon, in the name of Jesus.

42. Angel of God, protect me and my family, in the name of Jesus.

43. Every fowler snare, assign to capture my soul, break to pieces, in the name of Jesus.

44. Every arrow that flies by day, my life is not your candidate, backfire, in the name of Jesus.

45. Heavenly fire extinguisher, consume every disease around me, in the name of Jesus.

46. Fake fortress, fake refuge, assign to consume me, catch fire, and roast to ashes, in the name of Jesus.

47. I shall not strike my foot against stone of sickness and disease in the name of Jesus.

48. Wild lion assign to devour me, die, in the name of Jesus.

49. Serpent of sickness in my life, die in the name of Jesus.

50. I trample upon every serpent and scorpion delegated against me, in the name of Jesus.

51. Enough of sickness and disease, die and rise no more, in the name of Jesus.
52. Every disaster warming up to consume me, your time is up, die, in the name of Jesus.
53. Dark angels that manufacture and distribute killer disease, die in the name of Jesus.
54. O Lord, deliver me and honour me today, in the name of Jesus.
55. Dark shelter, prepared for me, catch fire and roast to ashes, in the name of Jesus.
56. O Lord my God, lay your hands of deliverance upon me, in the name of Jesus.
57. No disaster shall come near my household, in the name of Jesus.
58. No harm shall befall me and my family, in the name of Jesus.
59. At the end Lord, let salvation be my food and passport to heaven, in the name of Jesus.
60. A thousand of viruses may fly around, I shall not be affected, in the name of Jesus.
61. Ten thousand of sickness and disease may be released to consume souls, I shall not be affected, in the name of Jesus.
62. Disease around me shall die, and be like a day just gone by, in the name of Jesus.

63. Angels of God, sweep away what causes untimely death, I shall not be its portion, in the name of Jesus.

64. Spirit disease and infirmity around me, your time is up dry up, in the name of Jesus.

65. O Lord, do not allow your anger last long upon me, forgive me, and pity me, in the name of Jesus.

66. O Lord, let the length of my day on earth be long and not shorten by disease, in the name of Jesus.

67. O Lord, give me wisdom to handle situations around me in the name of Jesus.

68. O Lord, fill my heart with gladness, in the name of Jesus.

69. Every bondage holding me captive break in the name of Jesus.

70. I will serve my God and be blessed in the name of Jesus Amen

CHAPTER 3

PRAYER OF CLEANSING USING LUKE 4

Hope is not lost after all. The mighty may fall, but then there is hope, light will still shine at the end of the tunnel. Anger of God may come, with prayer, and supplication, he will listen and answer his chosen. God hates sin, he hates pride, and he hates all manners that don't promote his name.

We are to rise in prayer to him, to cleanse us of evil thought that make us victim of sickness and disease. Virus flies about because of our sins and deeds. Yet, he is ready to redeem us from the hands of the foe, virus that kills, infirmities that destroy, sickness that reduce one to nothing and disease that takes ones glory. People without heavenly cleansing are caught unaware and wandered about in agony. They wonder about with sickness of poverty, sickness of hatred and stagnation. They need healing to rise and shine, and this can only be, if they are cleansed.

In the book of Psalm, chapter 107 give details of affliction that arise for those who choose to dwell in sin. They find no way to settle. Spiritually they are clinically down and affected. Infirmity makes one hunger for healing; disease makes one thirst for good health. Plagues are all over causing infirmity and sickness to arrest and destroy souls. Such situation needs cleansing; cleansing of the soul and body. The question is, are you hungry and thirsty for heavenly cleansing? You shall cry out to the Lord Almighty to carry out clinical health operation in your life. Your body is not for sickness or disease. Cry unto him today for total cleansing and deliverance.

There are times we unknowingly sit in darkness, even in the deepest gloom. We clap hands, drink and dance, not knowing our life needs cleansing. It was like when plague break out in Egypt in the days of Moses, Pharaoh takes it for a joke. The Egyptians believed in there gods and never take Moses serious, until the night God passed over the land of Egypt and each Egyptian home lost their first born son. The plague came, it was like a flood. It swept the country down, cry and agony was the order of the day. The mighty fell and cry, old people in Egypt lost their balance and fell like packs of cards. Physicians in Egypt could not do anything. I pray no plague, sickness or disease shall visit your home.

The country needs hands of God upon them. Pharaoh the king was confuse. He wept bitterly, the land needs cleansing. Hundreds of first born died to the cold arm of death. Once again, the land needs cleansing, not until they let the Israelites go.

The bible says, **"Some became fools through their rebellious ways and suffered affliction because of their iniquities. They loathed all food and drew near the gates of death. Then they cried to the LORD in their trouble and he saved them from their distress" Psalm 107:17-19.** I pray, God shall listen to their cries and be saved from disaster.

Yes, God shall sent forth his word of healing unto us at large, and cleanse our land of every sickness, diseases and infirmities. Never shall we experience plague that will consume us. The world needs peace, no one needs plague.

The Lord shall proof HIMSELF. I AM that I AM shall appear in our lives. O Lord we all bow before you. Our GOD IS MIGHTY. Here we are O Lord, cleanse our land. We know you are in control. To you O LORD be the glory.

Let us arise now and pray.

PRAYER POINTS

1. I thank you Lord for the cleansing you will carry out in my life, in the name of Jesus.

2. I thank you Lord, for the clinical operation against disease in my life, in the name of Jesus.

3. I thank you Lord, infirmity shall not be my portion, in the name of Jesus.
4. I thank my God, for he is good, his love endures forever.
5. I thank my God, who redeem my soul, in the name of Jesus.
6. O Lord, forgive me sins that makes me distant from you, in the name of   Jesus.
7. O Lord, I bow before you, have mercy on me, in the name of Jesus.
8. Praise be to my God, who forgives my sin.
9. O Lord, forgive me, don't destroy me, in the name of Jesus.
10. O Lord, forgive the world of untimely death that occur as a result of sin.
11. Blood of Jesus, cleanse me of sickness living in my body, in the name of Jesus.
12. Blood of Jesus, cleanse me of any infirmity that may appear in my life, in the name of Jesus.
13. Blood of Jesus, purify my blood against any disease, in the name of Jesus.
14. I wash and cleanse my hands with heavenly sanitizer of God, in the name of Jesus.
15. Holy Spirit, break and destroy every plague in my environment, in the name of Jesus.

16. Holy Spirit, break every yoke in my life, in the name of Jesus.
17. Holy Spirit, guide me from every contamination that leads to death.
18. Holy Spirit, cleanse me, in the name of Jesus.
19. I am thirsty for heavenly cleansing, O Lord, cleanse me in the name of Jesus.
20. O Lord, visit me with power to heal and make me rise and shine, in the name of Jesus.
21. O Lord, redeem me from the hands of the foes, in the name of Jesus.
22. O Lord, save me from virus that kills, in the name of Jesus.
23. O Lord, save me from infirmities that kills, in the name of Jesus.
24. O Lord, save me from sickness that render one useless, in the name of Jesus.
25. O Lord arise in my defense, defend me from powers that kill glory, in the name of Jesus.
26. I shall not migrate to the hand of death, in the name of Jesus.
27. My body is not for disease, I reject you by fire, in the name of Jesus.
28. Lord Jesus, arise, carry out clinical operation in my body against sickness and disease, in the name of Jesus.

29. Light of God, shine in every dark I sit, in the name of Jesus.

30. Power of darkness, leave me alone, expire, in the name of Jesus.

31. O Lord, proof yourself for good upon us in the name of Jesus.

32. I shall not wonder away into the hand of cold death, in the name of Jesus.

33. Sudden death, the leveler, expire, in the name of Jesus.

34. I reject spirit that distributes sickness and disease, in the name of Jesus.

35. Broom of cleansing, sweep every killer to dustbin of death, in the name of Jesus.

36. O Lord, let peace reign in the world, in the name of Jesus.

37. Never again shall deadly disease, rise second time in the name of Jesus.

38. Satanic warfare against my nation, scatter in the name of Jesus.

39. Whatever the name of sickness or disease, it shall not be my portion in the name of Jesus.

40. O Lord, send forth your word of healing unto this land in the name of Jesus.

41. My cry to the Lord shall not be in vain, in the name of Jesus.

42. O Lord, save me from distress and confusion, in the name of Jesus.

43. O Lord, cleanse my spirit of rebellion to God, in the name of Jesus.

44. O Lord, heal our land in the name of Jesus.

45. When I sing unto the Lord (pick a song) my God shall heal me, in the name of Jesus.

46. When I clap hands unto the Lord, (clap your hand), my God shall heal me in the name of Jesus.

47. Heavenly doctor come to my life and cleanse me of any virus or disease, in the name of Jesus.

48. I shall not take what will kill me as joke in the name of Jesus.

49. Affliction shall not rise in my life, in the name of Jesus.

50. Disease of hatred and stagnation hunting my destiny your time is up, die, in the name of Jesus.

51. Poverty sickness assign to destroy my finance, expire, in the name of Jesus.

52. O Lord, I cry unto you for total cleansing and deliverance, help me, in the name of Jesus.

53. Where my life needs cleansing, I shall not play away in the name of Jesus.

54. Where my life needs cleansing, I shall not be rejected, in the name of Jesus.

55. I shall not weep over anyone in my family in the name of Jesus.

56. I shall not weep over my siblings in the name of Jesus.

57. I shall not lose my life to deadly epidemic in the name of Jesus.

58. Even I am taken to isolation centre, I will recover and be negative to virus in the name of Jesus.

59. I shall not be patient of isolation centre in the name of Jesus.

60. Powers that distribute sorrow shall not locate me, in the name of Jesus.

61. Agony shall not be my food, in the name of Jesus.

62. My body is not dedicated to disease, I reject your stay in my body, in the name of Jesus.

63. Our hope shall not be in vain, in the name of Jesus.

64. The mighty may fall and be victim I shall not be, in the name of Jesus.

65. My body is not dedicated to infirmity, I reject you by fire, in the name of Jesus.

66. I receive it, I am cleansed in the name of Jesus.

67. Heavenly cleansing angels of God, cleanse my body in the name of Jesus.
68. Heavenly cleansing angels of God, cleanse my environment, in the name of Jesus.
69. Heavenly cleansing angels of God, cleanse my soul, in the name of Jesus.
70. Heavenly cleansing angels of God, cleanse my home, in the name of Jesus. Amen

CHAPTER 4

PRAYER OF IMMUNITY USING ISAIAH 43

Immunity is what makes one not vulnerable to evil, disaster, attack, virus, disease and infirmity. When immune, you think of safety in the mind. Fear finds no place in your heart. It makes you feel right from danger.

Bullet proof cars immune the driver and occupants of gun shots. No matter the number of bullets fired on such car, it won't penetrate. Human beings in their wisdom produce such cars. But before then, God promised his children, you and me as well of spiritual proofs that safeguard life. In this regard, the book of Isaiah make us to understand there is fire proof, flood proof, water proof, even river proof of the Lord,. Here, we shall seek the Lord to equip us with air proof as well. This will protect us from virus disease that attack through the air. Virus is a disease you can't see with naked eyes. It is like a war with unseen powers. It is demon in the air, that arrest and kill people at will

The book of Isaiah is a book of promise from our creator and redeemer. The promise of God to redeem us is imminent. Hope is not lost if you are on the Lord's side. He said, "Fear not". This means you shall not be consumed by any form of sickness, infirmity or disease. Such are the handwork of Satan, which cannot override power of God.

Based on this, God said, **"When you pass through the waters, I will be with you, and when you pass through the rivers, they will not be burned, the flames will not set you ablaze. For I am the LORD, your God, the Holy One of Israel, your Saviour---" Isaiah 43:2-3.**

The God that said it then is still fresh alive! He is ageless and powerful, with Divine Power House of Wisdom. You are immune to problems, disaster, infirmity, and sickness and virus of any form. Why build fear in your mind, when God is there for you. Pray unto him for deliverance from seen and unseen powers

The Bible says, no water will consume you, when you pass through it. Forget about what the water has; call it marine power, serpentine marine power, deepness of the water, virus or disease of the water. You are safe! This is immunity. It says, no river shall sweep you away, meaning you can't be wiped away by any river, or be consumed by creatures in it. Mention it, hippopotamus, wild fish, crocodile, marine spirit, serpents; they won't harm or kill you. No matter how deep the river, its flow will not sweep you away. Why?, because the Lord is with you. This means no matter the name given to any water borne disease, you shall not be swallowed by it. No matter the danger of virus in rivers and waters, you shall not be a victim. Untimely death is not your portion. You are river proof and water proof of dangers.

Fire destroys with ease; it consumes whatever comes its way. Its flames cause havoc, it burns and destroys. But the Lord says, if he is with you, you won't be burned by fire! Ask the three Hebrew boys, they will tell you it is true. They even clap, dance and sing in the destructive flaming fire. God says, He is God of yesterday, today and indefinite tomorrow! You are fire proof, devoid of flame consumption. Do not fear of fire destructive weapons in the hands of disease, that kills at will globally. You are not its candidate, because the Lord is on your side.

The Holy One of Israel does not tell lies. He is ready to save you from the claws of dreaded powers, from the grip of spirit of death.

Surrender to Him today in prayer and in faith without fear. Let us pray and call upon him today.

PRAYER POINTS

1. I thank you O Lord, for your immunity upon my life, in the name of Jesus
2. I thank you my Lord, for your mercy upon me, in the name of Jesus
3. My thanksgiving goes to the Most High God, who care for me, in the name of Jesus
4. O Lord, I thank you for your love and favour for me, in the name of Jesus
5. Heavenly father, thank you as I see today again, in the name of Jesus
6. O Lord, forgive me the sins that may stand against me in my prayer today, in the name of Jesus
7. O Lord, naked every sin in me and disgrace them in my life, in the name of Jesus
8. O Lord, I bow down before you, forgive me known and unknown sins, in the name of Jesus
9. Doors of mercy and favour open unto me, in the name of Jesus

10. My hands be immune of sin, in the name of Jesus

11. I cover myself with immunity of the blood of Jesus

12. I soak myself in the pool blood of Jesus

13. I drink blood of Jesus to kill every strange thing in my body, in the name of Jesus

14. O Lord, let your blood be a mark on my forehead for protection against attacks of darkness in the name of Jesus

15. Holy Spirit Divine, immunize me against sickness and disease, in the name of Jesus

16. Holy Spirit, deliver me from attacks that leads to untimely death, in the name of Jesus

17. Holy Ghost Fire, consume powers assign to consume me, in the name of Jesus

18. O Lord, do new thing in my life today, in the name of Jesus

19. Every burden of disease waiting to consume me, catch fire and roast to ashes, in the name of Jesus.

20. O Lord my father, immunize me against sickness and disease in the name of Jesus

21. Promise of God upon my life, come to pass, in the name of Jesus

22. O Lord, make me great, in the name of Jesus

23. Spirit of righteousness, envelope my life in the name of Jesus
24. O Lord, give me spirit to pay attention of what surrounds me, in the name of Jesus
25. I shall not be trapped in the battle of sickness and disease in the name of Jesus.
26. I shall not be plundered or looted by virus disease, in the name of Jesus
27. Satanic virus shall not imprison me, in the name of Jesus
28. Virus of darkness, I send you back by fire, in the name of Jesus
29. Wicked virus, you shall not hand me over to untimely death in the name of Jesus
30. O Lord, let me obey the law of immunity and abide by it, in the name of Jesus
31. O Lord, wear me with garment of immunity, in the name of Jesus
32. I eat angelic food that boost immunity against sickness and disease, in the name of Jesus
33. Disease violence, do not come close to me, scatter in the name of Jesus
34. When I pass through fire, my God shall immunize me against flames of fire, in the name of Jesus

35. When I pass through the rivers, my God shall immunize me against attack, in the name of Jesus
36. When I pass through the waters, my God shall immunize me against attack, in the name of Jesus
37. I shall not be given in exchange to death, in the name of Jesus
38. Any disease competing with my glory, die, in the name of Jesus
39. My eyes shall not be blind to reality on ground, in the name of Jesus
40. My ears shall not be deaf to what will make me survive in life, in the name of Jesus
41. I shall dwell in the assembly of the living in the name of Jesus.
42. Any virus foretold shall not kill me, in the name of Jesus
43. Any reigning virus or disease where I live shall not consume me, in the name of Jesus
44. Satanic legal ground against my existence, scatter, in the name of Jesus
45. I am a chosen race of God, I shall not die untimely death, in the name of Jesus
46. God of ancient days, lay hand of healing upon me, in the name of Jesus

47. Every action taken against me in the spirit, be reversed, in the name of Jesus
48. I shall not be a hospital victim, in the name of Jesus
49. Every satanic reinforcement against me scatter, in the name of Jesus
50. My life shall not be snuffed out, in the name of Jesus.
51. Lord Jesus , immunize me from attack of darkness, in the name of Jesus
52. O Lord, I call upon you, make me whole, in the name of the Jesus
53. I shall not be a sacrificial lamb in the hands of enemy, in the name of Jesus
54. O Lord, blot out my transgression, so that I may enjoy your immunity in the name of Jesus
55. Every rebellion in my spirit, die, and rise no more, in the name of Jesus
56. Holy Ghost Power, consign every infirmity and disease to destruction, in the name of Jesus.
57. O Lord immunize me from thirst and destruction, in the name of Jesus
58. I shall dwell in the flowing streams of the Lord, and never be forsaken to destruction, in the name of Jesus
59. Every idol consulted to destroy me, catch fire and roast to ashes, in the name of Jesus

60. Every covenant of darkness against my life, break and backfire in the name of Jesus
61. Every witness raised to rob me of heavenly immunity scatter, in the name of Jesus
62. O Lord, remold me for signs and wonders, in the name of Jesus
63. Powers assign to scatter my destiny, be naked and powerless in the name of Jesus
64. O Lord, I cry unto you, listen to me and protect me, in the name of Jesus
65. Fire of God, come down and make me whole, in the name of Jesus
66. Power of infirmity upon my life, break, in the name of Jesus
67. I shall not be afraid, for the Lord is with me, in the name of Jesus
68. O Lord, gather my family together and immunize us against virus and diseases
69. O Lord, you created me for your glory, let my glory shine in the name of Jesus
70. I will not tremble or be afraid, my God is Yahweh, He shall save me, in the name of Jesus.

CHAPTER 5

PRAYER OF HOPE USING PSALM 41

Power and might is given by God. Power resides with God. He is Almighty God. Your muscle, height, race, intelligence and wisdom are not your creation, God deposited them in you. They are not your creation. God gives them for the betterment of his creation, Alas! We misfire and go about with pride. We regard others as nobody, we regard them as weak. When two, three or four nations struggle to outshine each other the grass will suffer.

Nations are on sick bed struggling for survival. There is no year one sickness, disease or infirmity is not mentioned. Even after the Ebola issue, mere mention of its name cause fear. There is another dreadful disease called corona virus that shakes the world to its foundation. The name is dreadful; it sends panic to everyone. Yet there is hope. The bible says, **"The LORD will sustain him on his sickbed and restore him from his bed of illness" Psalm 41:3.** This is hope for all.

Nations are counting losses, there is lockdown everywhere, stock prices fall and continue to fall, exchange rate soars, the weak are hungry and death rate multiplies.

Today, everybody seeks the face of God. Presidents, Prime Ministers, Queen and Kings are on their knee, crying to God, "Have mercy on us, have mercy on our nation O Lord". But then, hope is not lost. The Lord is there for us all, only if we sober, seek his face and surrender all to him.

The truth of the matter is, ordinary citizens don't know facts of this pandemic virus. World leaders make allegations against each other. There is allegation upon allegation. Here is the biblical equivalent to this, **"Whenever one comes to see me, he speaks falsely, while his heart gathers slander; then he goes out and spread it abroad" Psalm 41:6.** We are not happy with what is on ground. No one is happy with this situation, what we are saying is, "O Lord, our land needs healing"!

We are crying to God to heal the land, the earth and every home. The world must seek peace, we need it. We don't want sickness, disease or infirmity, the land needs healing. **"All my enemies whisper together against me; they imagine the worst for me, saying, "A vile disease has beset him; he will never get up from the place where he lies" Psalm41:7-8.** This is the boast of the enemy.

The Lord is there for us. We must go back to him for hope (healing), to materialize. "O Lord, show mercy upon us, we trust you can do it" This is what we should have in mind. It is when we surrender all, God will listen to us. There is hope; all will be well. Dangers inherent in COVID-19 shall expire, lamentation of the earth shall receive answer, death toll shall soon reach zero level, families shall smile, wickedness of the wicked shall end. Our hope shall not be dashed to pieces. Amen.

Now let's pray.

PRAYER POINTS

1. O Lord, forgive our nation of her pride, in the name of Jesus.
2. O Lord, forgive me and others of pride, in the name of Jesus.
3. O Lord, forgive us of our wickedness, in the name of Jesus.
4. O Lord, forgive every nation of their sins, in the name of Jesus.
5. I thank you Lord for not bringing this earth to end, in the name of Jesus
6. I thank you Lord, for your mercy upon our land, in the name of Jesus.

7. I thank you Lord, for opening door of hope to us, in the name of Jesus.

8. I thank you Lord, for the healing of our land you are doing right now, in the name of Jesus.

9. I thank you Lord, for you wipe away our sorrow, in the name of Jesus.

10. Blood of Jesus, heal our land, in the name of Jesus.

11. I drink blood of Jesus to purify my body in the name of Jesus.

12. I drink blood of Jesus, to immunize my spirit, soul and body in the name of Jesus.

13. I drink blood of Jesus, to improve my hope in the name of Jesus.

14. I cover myself with blood of Jesus to serve as protection against attack, in the name of Jesus.

15. Holy Spirit, guide our steps, this day in the name of Jesus.

16. Holy Spirit, speak to our soul to do good, in the name of Jesus.

17. Holy Ghost Power, fight the battle we can't see, in the name of Jesus.

18. Holy Ghost, touch every heart planning to harm the earth, in the name of Jesus.

19. Every virus spreading to bring my house down shall fail in the name of Jesus.

20. Every virus manufactured to destroy the world, die in the name of Jesus.
21. My hope shall not be dashed as a result of virus flying around, in the name of Jesus.
22. Lord Jesus, kill killer spirit troubling the world, in the name of Jesus.
23. O Lord, let your grace be sufficient for me, in the name of Jesus.
24. My hope shall not be extinguished by enemy in the name of Jesus.
25. Every secret to harm this world be exposed, in the name of Jesus.
26. I claim victory over satanic agenda, in the name of Jesus.
27. Virus power competing with my success, expire, in the name of Jesus.
28. O Lord, bring to an end pride in the life of people creating proplems in the name of Jesus.
29. O Lord, heal nations on sick bed, in the name of Jesus.
30. By his stripe, every nation shall be healed, in the name of Jesus.
31. Power and effect of sickness and disease expire, in the name of Jesus.
32. Power and effect of flu in every nation expire, in the name of Jesus.

33. Power and effect of corona virus in every nation expire, in the name of Jesus.
34. Power and effect of infirmities upon my life expire, in the name of Jesus.
35. Power and effect of bad health upon my life expire, in the name of Jesus.
36. Disease and infirmity that sicken the world expire, in the name of Jesus.
37. O Lord, restore everyone on sickbed to life, in the name of Jesus.
38. I shall not count losses as a result of infirmity, in the name of Jesus.
39. Virus that causes lock down expire, in the name of Jesus.
40. Virus that bring trades to its kneel; expire, in the name of Jesus.
41. I shall not be weak or hungry, in the name of Jesus.
42. Sickness and diseases that causes death expire in the name of Jesus.
43. Powers spreading bad news about me be disgraced to nothing, in the name of Jesus.
44. Powers spreading bad news about my nation be disgraced to nothing, in the name of Jesus.
45. Hope killers in the world, my God shall judge you, in the name of Jesus.

46. Hope killers in my country, my God shall judge you, in the name of Jesus.
47. Hope killers in my environment, my God shall judge you, in the name of Jesus.
48. Agenda of darkness for me and my household scatter in the name of Jesus.
49. My foundation, receive healing in the name of Jesus.
50. Every attack against my foundation scatter, in the name of Jesus.
51. Every wickedness of the wicked against my soul backfire, in the name of Jesus.
52. Enemies of my soul, become powerless, in the name of Jesus.
53. Evil garment prepared for me catch fire and roast to ashes, in the name of Jesus.
54. Powers fighting me because of the riches of my country be disgraced, in the name of Jesus.
55. Every nation fighting my country in cold war, be exposed and be impotent, in the name of Jesus.
56. Our land need healing, O Lord heal it, in the name of Jesus.
57. Fire of God; consume epidemic assign to devour us, in the name of Jesus.
58. Every coalition to trouble the world scatters, in the name of Jesus.

59. Those that imagine worst for me shall fail in the name of Jesus.

60. O Lord, we surrender all to you, have mercy on us, in the name of Jesus.

61. O Lord, we seek your face, answer us, in the name of Jesus.

62. O Lord, give me power to forge ahead, in the name of Jesus.

63. O Lord, let my nation sing songs of melody and joy, in the name of Jesus.

64. O Lord, let songs of melody fill my mouth in the name of Jesus.

65. No weapon fashioned against my nation shall prosper, in the name of Jesus.

66. No weapon fashioned against my soul shall prosper, in the name of Jesus.

67. O Lord, pour anointing of healing upon my life, in the name of Jesus.

68. I decree restoration of greatness upon my life in the name of Jesus.

69. Power of greatness, locate me by fire, in the name of Jesus.

70. Prophetic announcement for my life manifest, in the name of Jesus.

CHAPTER 6

PRAYER OF ASSURANCE USING EXODUS 15

The Israelites get to Marah after hectic walk of three days of thirsty. The water they found was bitter, they could not drink it. The situation of the world can be described as Marah. The world is full of bitterness. There is bitterness among nations, there is racial conflict and bitterness, and there is power tussle of bitterness as well.

Such bitterness made nations outdo themselves, it affects the world. Biological weapons are produced, tested and exposed to innocent citizens. This led to virus export. The case of corona virus fit in here, where many families are in agony. Sorrow became their food. Heart attack was prominent. High blood pressure takes over normal body temperature leading to high blood pressure. There is cry upon cry. Cries take over the land. Doctors were not spared, they died in hundred. It was as if nurses were main target. They died in multiples. What of other health workers?, untimely death visit them and devour them like biscuits in the mouth of children. This I may call global Marah. It is so pathetic. The scene is ugly.

The Marah time came to play in the book of Exodus chapter 15, shortly when the Israelites crossed the Red Sea; they put trust in the Lord, and sang songs of hope and assurance. **"Then Miriam the prophetess, Aaron's sister, took a tambourine in her hand, and all the women followed her, with tambourines and dancing" Exodus 15:20.**

This is replica of the situation before Ebola, and or, COVID 19 strikes. There was joy before they appeared. Once they appeared, the disease changed the template of existence. Marah or sadness appeared, the center could not hold. We grumble in the order of Israelites. **"So the people grumbled against Moses" Exodus 15:24.**

Moses cried out to the Lord and the Lord answered. This gives me assurance, if we cry to God, He will answer us. Every Marah shall disappear in our life, in our neighborhood and the world at large. Why, because the virus is manmade. Those behind it are not above God. The Lord will arise to the situation and silence it. Let's build hope, raise faith and put everything under control. It shall be eliminated. The Lord cures and shall raise people that will silence the deadly virus from doing more havoc to human race.

There is assurance that God will answer our prayer. There is assurance that the ancient of days shall answer us by fire. There is assurance that powers of darkness shall bow to heavenly pressure and command. There is assurance that we shall soon smile. There is assurance that failure will not be our portion. There is assurance that sickness and disease shall not be our portion or stagnate us. There is assurance we shall live above virus and infirmities.

This is the reason, God assured the Israelites, "----**I will not bring on you any of the diseases I brought on the Egyptians, for I am the LORD, who heals you" Exodus 15:26.** Virus is a mother of disease. Sickness and disease graduate to kill. Disease sinks homes and brings disaster to family and nation. Many countries are under lockdown during corona virus epidemic. People are sober, but the Lord says, don't fear, I shall heal thee".

Every assurance from God shall be fulfilled. He doesn't tell lies. He affirms his words. He takes action at appropriate time, if we call him. He is there for us. We need to pray, to bring down his hand of healing we need God's presence in our lives. No one can do it, except God.

To bring the assurance to light and experience his hand of healing, we shall pray. Let's go into season of prayer with double assurance. It is time to pray.

PRAYER POINTS

1. I thank you Lord for you shall bring assurance of fulfillment to my life, in the name of Jesus.
2. I thank my God, who shall listen to my prayer and answer me, in the name of Jesus.
3. I thank my God for his assurance is genuine and accurate.
4. I thank God for his love for me, in the name of Jesus.
5. I thank my God for his majesty, in the name of Jesus.
6. O Lord, forgive me of my sins, in the name of Jesus.
7. O Lord, let your forgiveness be total upon my life, in the name of Jesus.
8. O Lord, I cry for total forgiveness that open great door of good health to life, do it for me, in the name of Jesus.
9. Every sin working against my health, expire, by the power in the name of Jesus.
10. I drink blood of Jesus to purify my body, in the name of Jesus.

11. I wash myself in the pool blood of Jesus.

12. Blood of Jesus be a mark of "Virus, disease and sickness quit my child" in my life in the name of Jesus.

13. Holy Spirit, pour blood of Jesus upon my head, to flow from my head to my toes, in the name of Jesus.

14. I shall not sink in life; Holy Spirit shall lift me above deadly disease, in the name of Jesus.

15. O Lord, feed me with Holy Communion that kills virus and disease.

16. Holy Ghost power, turn my life around, in the name of Jesus.

17. Holy Ghost fire, burn every virus attach to my body, in the name of Jesus.

18. Holy Ghost power, lay hand of healing upon me, in the name of Jesus.

19. Water of Marah in my life, dry up in the name of Jesus.

20. Marah water of disease, dry up in the name of Jesus.

21. Every water in my life, assign to cause untimely death dry up in the name of Jesus.

22. Divine water of God, boil to high temperature, and kill virus that attack souls worldwide, in the name of Jesus.

23. Every dark water in my body, assisting sickness and disease to grow in my life dry up, in the name of Jesus.

24. Thirsty disease assign to kill the cells in my body, so that I experience untimely death, die, in the name of Jesus.

25. Racial conflicts that lead to generation of deadly disease scatter, in the name of Jesus.

26. Biological weapon operating in the world be silenced by hands of God, in the name of Jesus.

27. O Lord, scatter the plan of countries planning evil against my country, in the name of Jesus.

28. Heart attack as a result of sickness and disease, expire in the name of Jesus.

29. High blood pressures, as a result of sickness and disease, expire in the name of Jesus.

30. My family shall not fall victim of disease and infirmity in the name of Jesus.

31. O Lord, empower me to have quiet time with you in the name of Jesus.

32. Virus, disease and infirmity in my environment die in the name of Jesus.

33. I cry to you O Lord, answer me in the name of Jesus.

34. River Marah, flowing against my health dry up in the name of Jesus.

35. River Marah flowing against my destiny dry up, in the name of Jesus.
36. River Marah flowing to feed my body with sickness, dry up, in the name of Jesus.
37. River Marah around me disappear, in the name of Jesus.
38. My home shall not be under lockdown to disease and infirmity, in the name of Jesus.
39. Power of lockdown over my nation, expire in the name of Jesus.
40. Every hope and assurance of God for my life be fulfilled, in the name of Jesus.
41. Powers behind corona virus be put to shame, expire, in the name of Jesus.
42. Manmade virus, die, in the name of Jesus.
43. Power of darkness, distributing virus, my life is not your candidate, expire, in the name of Jesus.
44. Disease and infirmity shall not stagnate me, in the name of Jesus.
45. Virus shall not sink my home, in the name of Jesus.
46. Disaster shall not locate my family in the name of Jesus.
47. Hand of healing from above be upon my head for total deliverance of good health, in the name of Jesus.

48. I shall not fear but be strong in the Lord, in the name of Jesus.

49. I shall not die but live, in the name of Jesus.

50. Every assurance of God upon me shall be fulfilled, in the name of Jesus.

51. My destiny be converted from sorrow to happiness, in the name of Jesus.

52. Agony shall not be my portion in the name of Jesus.

53. My mouth shall not push me to sin, in the name of Jesus.

54. Curative powers of God come upon me in the name of Jesus.

55. Thou deadly disease causing havoc to human race, die, in the name of Jesus.

56. O Lord, decorate me with garment of good health in the name of Jesus.

57. Failure will not be my portion in the name of Jesus.

58. O Lord arise, raise people that will eliminate every disease tormenting the world, in the name of Jesus.

59. Songs of assurance fill my mouth in the name of Jesus.

60. Songs of hope fill my mouth, in the name of Jesus.

61. Songs of deliverance and health breakthrough fill my mouth in the name of Jesus.
62. Satanic padlock assign to lock my health, break in the name of Jesus.
63. Sickness and disease shall not stagnate me in the name of Jesus.
64. Thou power of darkness, bow to heavenly control in the name of Jesus.
65. O Lord, fill my mouth with heavenly smiles in the name of Jesus.
66. My house shall not receive sorrow as visitor in the name of Jesus.
67. My tambourine of good health, locate me and broadcast the mightiness of God in my life, in the name of Jesus.
68. I shall live above virus and infirmity, in the name of Jesus.
69. No virus, sickness, disease or infirmity shall consume me, in the name of Jesus.
70. Assurance of God upon me to live long and not die untimely death shall prevail upon my life, in the name of Jesus.

CHAPTER 7

PRAYER FOR FAMILY, NEIGHBOUR AND NATIONS

Nations are made up of diverse families. A home is a fragment part of a nation. An individual is a citizen of a nation. Each family form a home, around them are other homes, called neighbours. These are home neighbours. Wherever you work, or reside you will have neighbours whether you interact or not. In office, in the bus, in the farm, church or mosque, whoever is with you or around you is your neighbour.

Family expands to form neighbours, neighbours in large geographical location form a nation. They are close ties, that can't be separated. Whatever affects families, affects the nation. Disease outbreak can start in a family, if not curbed; it will affect neighbours around them and spread within the nation. Hence, an atom becomes mountain to contend with. **"When the foundations are being destroyed, what can the righteous do?" Psalm 11:3.** The righteous will be affected if correct step is not taken.

If infirmity or disease encroach a home, it should not be taken lightly. It must be handled with care and love, or else, it will spread and infect others. Thereby, spread from arithmetic to geometric progression. The best, is to nip it in the bud.

Your family needs healing, your neighbour needs healing, your nation needs healing as well. The nation is the head, and when the head is sick, the body; that is, family and neighbours, sick as well. Corona virus started in Wahun, it spread across international borders and inflicted nations. Ebola started in Africa, it shakes the world. HIV/AIDS started from individual. It spread like wild fire and threaten health system.

For this reason, we must pray to set our family free of diseases and sickness. We must pray for our neighbour's freedom from the grip of virus, sickness and disease. We must arise and pray for our nation. The time is now, we must not tarry.

Now let's pray.

PRAYER FOR FAMILY

1. I thank you Lord for your protection upon my family in the name of Jesus.

2. I thank you Lord, that no soul shall lost in my family to sickness or disease in the name of Jesus.

3. O Lord forgive my family of ancestral and present sins hunting our lineage, in the name of Jesus.

4. I cover my family with blood of Jesus, from pit of hell, in the name of Jesus.

5. Blood of Jesus, cancel evil report against my family, in the name of Jesus.

6. Holy Ghost fire sanitize my family line in the name of Jesus.

7. Where is the Lord God of Elijah, arise, heal my family of any sickness or disease in the name of Jesus.

8. Power of deliverance, locate my family for healing in the name of Jesus.

9. Desert spirit in my lineage, die, in the name of Jesus.

10. Satanic arrangement assign to bombard my family with disease and infirmity scatter, in the name of Jesus.

11. Strong wind of the Lord, blow against virus and diseases assign to harm my family in the name of Jesus.

12. Every stone of darkness thrown into my family to cause havoc, backfire, in the name of Jesus.

13. Any illness energizing failure at the edge of breakthrough in my family, expire, in the name of Jesus.
14. Every problem that come into my family, expire, in the name of Jesus.
15. Every enemy of my health, become impotent, in the name of Jesus.
16. Every marine spirit assign to pollute my health, die, in the name of Jesus.
17. Every sickness projected into my family, expire, in the name of Jesus.
18. Night caterer assign to feed my family with satanic food so that I fall sick and die, be disgraced, in the name of Jesus.
19. Yoke of bad health in my family line, break, in the name of Jesus.
20. Evil chain of darkness holding the health of my family captive, break in the name of Jesus.
21. Satanic virus in my family line, die, in the name of Jesus.
22. Bareness as a result of disease and sickness that takes me hostage, die, in the name of Jesus.
23. I release my family from witchcraft cage, in the name of Jesus.
24. I fire back every arrow of sickness and disease fired against my family, in the name of Jesus.

25. My family shall not waste finance on sickness in the name of Jesus.

26. Any damage done to my family through sickness and disease, be healed in the name of Jesus.

27. O Lord, incubate my family for good health and success in the name of Jesus.

28. I speak destruction, to every mountain of health challenges, in the name of Jesus.

29. Father Lord, correct anything that is wrong in my family in the name of Jesus.

30. O Lord give my family miracle testimonies, in the name of Jesus.

PRAYER FOR NEIGHBOURS

1. O Lord, I thank you for your protection upon my neighbour, in the name of Jesus.
2. I thank you Lord, the number of my neighbour shall not decrease, in the name of Jesus.
3. Lord Jesus, lay hand of forgiveness upon my neighbour.
4. Rain of forgiveness, pour upon my neighbour in the name of Jesus.
5. Holy Spirit Divine, guide and protect my neighbour in the name of Jesus.
6. Holy Ghost power, declare good things into the lives of my neighbour, in the name of Jesus.
7. O Lord, fight against them that fight against my neighbour in the name of Jesus.
8. Every yoke of sickness and disease troubling my neighbour, break, in the name of Jesus.
9. O Lord, set my neighbour free from every sickness and disease, in the name of Jesus.
10. Violent angels of God, guide my neighbour, day and night in the name of Jesus.
11. Satanic wind blowing against my neighbour stop by fire, in the name of Jesus.
12. All curses and spells, working against my neighbour, break, in the name of Jesus.

13. Every power of wickedness in charge of the destiny of my neighbours, expire, in the name of Jesus.

14. Every artillery of disease and sickness against my neighbours, backfire, in the name of Jesus.

15. Every secret I need to know about my environment, be revealed, in the name of Jesus.

16. Every band of wickedness over my environment, scatter in the name of Jesus.

17. Every dream of sickness and disease, hunting my neighbours, your time is up, scatter, in the name of Jesus.

18. Environmental witchcraft controlling the affairs of my neighbours expire, in the name of Jesus.

19. Witchcraft agenda for my neighbours scatter, in the name of Jesus.

20. O Lord give my neighbours wing of great eagle to escape attack of virus and disease, in the name of Jesus.

21. O God arise, pronounce healing upon my neighbours in the name of Jesus.

22. Let shower of blessing pour down upon my neighbours in the name of Jesus.

23. Voice of Satan against my neighbours, be nullified in the name of Jesus.

24. Altar of affliction set up against my neighbour, catch fire and roast to ashes in the name of Jesus.

25. My neighbour shall not experience evil clinical prophecy in the name of Jesus.

26. My neighbours receive your miracle, in the name of Jesus.

27. O Lord, let your anointing flow upon my neighbours in the name of Jesus.

28. O Lord, lay your healing hands upon my neighbours in the name of Jesus.

29. Let the embargo upon my neighbours, break and scatter in the name of Jesus.

30. O Lord, I thank you, for your mercy, love, fruitfulness and breakthrough upon my neighbours in the name of Jesus.

PRAYER FOR THE NATION

1. I thank you Lord for your mercy upon my country, in the name of Jesus.
2. I thank you Lord, for counting my country worthy, in the name of Jesus.
3. O Lord, forgive my country of our sins in the name of Jesus.
4. O Lord, let your love for my nation, overshadow her sins, in the name of Jesus.
5. Blood of Jesus, cover my nation against evil carrier of virus, in the name of Jesus.
6. Holy Ghost fire, sanitize my nation of sickness and disease in the name of Jesus.
7. Every country that wants my country to be on the ground without strength to breakthrough, scatter, in the name of Jesus.
8. Satanic foundation of sickness and disease in my country, be uprooted in the name of Jesus.
9. Every bank of sickness and disease assign for my nation, catch fire and roast to ashes, in the name of Jesus.
10. O Lord, deliver the soul of my country from the wicked, in the name of Jesus.
11. O Lord bring the conspiracy of other nations against my country to nothing in the name of Jesus.

12. Every lying tongue against my country, paralyze, in the name of Jesus.
13. When enemies encamp against my nation, they shall scatter, in the name of Jesus.
14. Powers assign to embarrass the health of my nation, your time is up, expire, in the name of Jesus.
15. Fire of God, cleanse every disease in my country, in the name of Jesus.
16. Every register and calendar of darkness in my country, catch fire and roast to ashes, in the name of Jesus.
17. O Lord, let the rage of sickness and disease in my country expire, in the name of Jesus.
18. Demonic monitoring gadget supervising my country, be pulled down, in the name of Jesus.
19. Any material or object used to monitor my country become useless in the name of Jesus.
20. O Lord, fight against the destroyer working against the increase of my country, in the name of Jesus.
21. O Lord my father, deliver my country from generational health hazard, in the name of Jesus.
22. O Lord, let every sickness and disease troubling my nation, die, in the name of Jesus.

23. Anything planted in my country, fighting spirit of good health, you are a failure, wither and die, in the name of Jesus.

24. Eaters of flesh and drinkers of blood in my country, your time is up, scatter to desolation, in the name of Jesus.

25. Evil that held my country down, catch fire and roast to ashes, in the name of Jesus.

26. O Lord, deliver my nation from powers stronger than her, in the name of Jesus.

27. Evil association that gather in my country to pollute the air and cause havoc, scatter in the name of Jesus.

28. My country, claim prophecy of clinical good health, in the name of Jesus.

29. Father Lord, let my country multiply in good health, in the name of Jesus.

30. O Lord, make covenant of peace with this nation in the name of Jesus.

YOU HAVE BATTLES TO WIN
TRY THESE BOOKS

1. COMMAND THE DAY.

Each day of the week is loaded with meanings and divine assurance. God did not create each day of the week for the fun of it. Blessings, success, gifts, resources, hopes, portfolios, duties, rights, prophecies, warnings and challenges, are loaded in each day.

Do you know the language, command or decree you can use to claim what belongs to you in each day of the week? Do you know in Christendom, Monday can be equated to one of the days of creation in Genesis chapter one? Do you know creation lasted for six days and God rested on the seventh day? What day of the week can Christian equate as the first day of the week, if we follow Christian calendar? What day can we call day seven?

This book shall give insight to these questions. It shall explain how you can command each day of the week according to creation in the book of Genesis chapter one.

Above all, you shall exercise your right and claim what is hidden in each day of the week.
Check for this in **COMMAND THE DAY.**

2. PRAYER TO REMEMBER DREAMS

A lot of people are passing through this spiritual epidemic on a daily basis. Their dream life is epileptic, having no ability to remember all dreams they dream, or sometimes forget everything entirely. This is nothing but spiritual havoc you need to erase from your spiritual record.

The answer to every form of spiritual blackout caused by spiritual erasers is found in, **PRAYER TO REMEMBER DREAMS.**

3.100% CONFESSSIONS AND PROPHECIES TO LOCATE HELPERS.

This is a wonderful book on confessions and prophecies to locate helpers and helpers to locate you. It is a prayer book loaded with over two thousand (2,000) prayer points.

The book unravels how to locate unknown helpers, prayers to arrest mind of helpers and prayers for manifestation after encounter with helpers.

4. ANOINTING FOR ELEVENTH HOUR HELP.

This book tells much of what to do at injury hour called eleventh hour. When you read and use this book as prescribed fear shall vanish in your life when pursuing a project, career or contract.

5. PRAYER TO LOCATE HELPERS.

Our divine helper is God. He created us to be together and be of help to one another. In the midst of no help we lost out, ending our journey in the wilderness.

There are keys assign to open right doors of life. You need right key to locate your helpers. Enough is enough; of suffering in silence.

With this book, you shall locate your helpers while your helpers shall locate you.

6. FIRE FOR FIRE PRAYER BOOK

This prayer book is fast at answering spiritual problems. It is a bulldozer prayer book, full of prayers all through. It is highly recommended for night vigil. Testimonies are pouring in daily from users of this book across the world!

7. PRAYER FOR THE FRUIT OF THE WOMB

This prayer book is children magnet. By faith and believe in God Almighty, as soon as you use this book open doors to child bearing shall be yours. Amen

8. PRAYER FOR PREGNANT WOMEN.

This is a spiritual prayer book loaded with prayers of solution for pregnant women. As soon as you take in, the prayers you shall pray from day one of conception to the day of delivery are written in this book.

9. WARFARE IN THE OFFICE

It is high time you pray prayers of power must change hands in office. Use this book and liberate yourself from every form of office yoke.

10. MY MARRIAGE SHALL NOT BREAK

Marriage is corner piece of life, happiness and joy. You need to hold it tight and guide it from wicked intruders and destroyer of homes.

11. VICTORY OVER SATANIC HOUSE 1 & 2

Are you a tenant, Land lord bombarded left and right, front and back by wicked people around you?

With this book you shall be liberated from the hooks of the enemy.

12. DICTIONARY OF DREAMS

This is a must book for every home. It gives accurate details to about **10,000 (Ten thousand) dreams and interpretations,** written in alphabetical order for quick reference and easy digestion. The book portrays spiritual revelations

with sound prophetic guidelines. It is loaded with Biblical references and violent prayers.
Ask for yours today.

For Further Enquiries Contact
THE AUTHOR
EVANGELIST TELLA OLAYERI
P.O. Box 1872 Shomolu Lagos.
Tel: 08023583168

FROM AUTHOR'S DESK

BEFORE YOU GO

Hello,

Thank you for purchasing this book. Would you consider posting a review about this book? In addition to providing feedback and arousing others into Christ's bosom, reviews can help other customers to know about the book.

Please take a minute to leave a review on this book.

I would appreciate that!

Thank you in advance, for your review and your patronage!!

NOTE: You can get all my books from my website www.tellaolayeri.com

GOOD NEWS!!!

My audiobook is now available, to get one visit acx.com and search **"Tella Olayeri."**

Brethren, to be loaded and reloaded visit: *amazon.com/author/tellaolayeri* for a full spiritual sojourn for my books.

Thanks.

www.ingramcontent.com/pod-product-compliance
Lightning Source LLC
Chambersburg PA
CBHW070754250726
48662CB00004B/1790